Complementary Therapies for Body and Mind

Magaly Díaz Barrios

ISBN: 9798325251559

Copyright © 2024 Book "Complementary Therapies for Body and Mind"

Author: Magaly Diaz Barrios.

All rights reserved. Reproduction, distribution, or transmission of this book in any form or by any means, electronic, photocopying, or recording, without the author's consent, is prohibited.

Dedication

To my son Camilo for being the driving force

behind my world, to continue on this

beautiful journey of life.

Acknowledgments

First of all, thanks to the Father's energy that always accompanies me, illuminating my daily life.

To my son Camilo, for always supporting me with my projects and giving me so much love.

To all the professionals in the areas described in this book for their teachings, which have somehow served me in the advancement of health.

Index

Within the pages of this book, **"Complementary Therapies for Body and Mind,"** I share various paths that lead to improvement, healing, and balance of the mind and body.

After facing the challenge of breast cancer on two occasions, I document here everything I have undertaken to restore my body, marked by the aftermath of radiotherapy and chemotherapy. Additionally, through testimonials, I have witnessed how people have overcome different illnesses through complementary medicines and therapies. There are multiple forms and methods to emerge victorious from the traces left by various diseases. I confess that fear was present on many occasions, not because of death itself, but because of the suffering of experiencing something adverse again. The aftermath was tough to resolve, but the burning desire to live on this earth with a healthy body and mind was my driving force.

This process has been beautiful, allowing me to discover methods and practices that I never imagined. These tools have been crucial to explore my identity, make significant changes, and learn to strengthen both my body and mind.

In these pages, I propose comparative analyses to better understand our body and coordinate actions with our mind to achieve a quicker and more effective balance.

I invite you to choose those practices that resonate with you. Discipline is fundamental, but even more important are the desire and perseverance you put into it. If you truly desire a healthy and vital body, remember that "constancy overcomes what joy cannot reach".

Everything I present in this book is to offer you a glimpse of the complementary therapies available to assist our bodies. I am not a healthcare professional; I have only taken courses and seminars in search of answers to questions such as why illnesses persist in my body after cancer, such as Sjögren's syndrome, severe vertigo, and gastrointestinal problems. My insistence and perseverance have allowed me to improve more each day.

Today, some of these practices I perform by myself, thanks to the knowledge gained about my body and mind.

Chapter 1

Speaking of Ayurveda

> "A balanced diet nourishes
> both the body and the soul"

Ayurveda, known as the "science of life," consists of ancient wisdom for achieving a balanced life through natural remedies and lifestyle changes. Originating from India and practiced for thousands of years, Ayurveda offers numerous benefits for addressing various illnesses and improving quality of life. Instead of focusing solely on disease, this medical system aims to treat the patient as a whole, in harmony with disease prevention by cleansing the body and restoring balance between the body, mind, and spirit.

Ayurvedic Medicine encompasses strict dietary practices, medicinal herbs, exercises, meditation, physiotherapy, and other methods that have shown significant benefits in alleviating symptoms in patients with various conditions such as stress, anxiety, joint pain, insomnia, migraines, Parkinson's, fibromyalgia, Alzheimer's, asthma, high blood pressure, and arthritis.

Ayurvedic Medicine not only addresses discomfort but also focuses on addressing underlying causes, taking into account the patient's emotional and mental state, habits, environment, and climate. Furthermore, this natural and traditional therapeutic system complements allopathic medicine and was recognized by the World Health Organization for its value in disease treatment.

This therapy holds that all disorders of the body originate in people's minds, manifesting in organ or psychic disorders. It emphasizes that human well-being depends not only on physical health and the absence of disease but also on the balance of the mind, spirit, and social aspects. Ayurvedic medicine serves three fundamental functions: preventive, psychological, and curative.

In Ayurveda, six stages of disease are recognized, known as "Kriyakala" These stages represent the progression of the disease from its initial manifestations to its full manifestation. Here is a description of each of the stages:

1. **Initial Symptoms:** In this stage, imbalances in the doshas begin to accumulate in the body, but symptoms are not yet evident. The person may experience mild discomfort

or subtle changes in health, but may not necessarily recognize that something is wrong.

2. **Aggravation**: In this stage, dosha imbalances increase and begin to manifest more clearly. Symptoms become more evident, and the person starts to notice significant changes in their health.

3. **Accumulation**: During this stage, specific symptoms of the disease begin to manifest more clearly. For example, if the disease affects the respiratory system, the person may experience persistent cough, difficulty breathing, or other symptoms related to the lungs.

4. **Localization**: In this phase, the disease becomes localized in a specific area of the body. Symptoms concentrate on a particular organ or system, and the disease begins to impact the function and health of that specific area.

5. **Manifestation**: In this stage, the disease fully manifests with all its symptoms and effects. The person clearly experiences the full impact of the disease on their body and health.

6. **Diversification**: In this advanced stage, the disease may begin to cause complications and side effects in other

areas of the body, leading to the emergence of multiple symptoms and health problems.

These stages represent how the disease progresses and manifests in the body and mind, according to the Ayurvedic perspective. The goal of treatment in Ayurveda is to identify and treat the disease in the early stages to prevent its progression to more advanced stages.

The Dhatus and their objectives.

To complete the circle of holistic balance, it is essential to understand the "dhatus" of the body, which represent the seven bodily tissues: plasma, blood, muscle, fat, bone, bone marrow or nerve, and reproductive tissue.

The aim is to understand the dhatus, as when we ingest something, it is distributed to the different types of dhatus.

1. **Plasma refers** to the body's primary fluids and is essential for maintaining the quality and quantity of water in each person's body.

2. **Blood** is composed of fire and water, is fluid, and transports heat, ensuring cell oxygenation. Lack of oxygen in cells can lead to diseases such as cancer.

3. **Muscle** is predominantly earth with water and fire, forms a significant part of the body, and provides strength to the basic body structure, providing courage, confidence, and strength when in good condition.

4. **Fat** is mainly composed of water, serves lubrication functions in muscles, tendons, and other tissues, contributing to a more melodious voice by lubricating the throat.

5. **Bone**, primarily composed of minerals representing the earth, is capable of regeneration and provides strong support for tissues and organs, providing courage, confidence, and security when in good condition.

6. **Marrow and Nerves** are subtle parts of water, playing an important role in transmitting nerve impulses, as well as lubricating the eyes, stool, and skin, filling the empty spaces of the body.

7. **Reproductive Fluid** is the essential form of water that has the power to create new life. Its insufficiency can cause loss of creativity, infertility, and impotence.

In traditional Indian medicine, six distinct tastes are recognized to have an effect on energy and balance in the body. Each taste is associated with different elements and properties, and consuming a balanced combination of these tastes is believed to help maintain harmony in the body and mind.

The 6 Tastes

1. **Sweet**: This taste is associated with earth and water and is found in foods such as rice, milk, wheat, ripe fruits, and vegetables like carrots and sweet potatoes. The sweet taste is considered nourishing, soothing, and satisfying.

2. **Sour**: This taste is associated with fire and is found in foods such as yogurt, vinegar, lemon, and certain acidic fruits. The sour taste is believed to stimulate appetite and digestion.

3. **Salty**: This taste is associated with water and is found in foods such as salt, seaweed, and certain vegetables. The salty taste is considered hydrating and can balance the excess of other flavors in the diet.

4. **Spicy**: This taste is associated with fire and air and is found in foods such as chili, garlic, ginger, and some spices. The spicy taste is believed to stimulate digestion and metabolism.

5. **Bitter**: This taste is associated with ether and air and is found in foods such as arugula, turmeric, dark chocolate, and coffee. The bitter taste is considered purifying and detoxifying.

6. **Astringent**: This taste is associated with air and earth and is found in foods such as legumes, apples, Brussels sprouts, and certain herbs. The astringent taste is believed to have anti-inflammatory properties and can help tone tissues.

These tastes are important in Ayurveda, and consuming a balanced combination of them is believed to contribute to harmony in the body and mind.

With proper nutrition according to each individual's dosha, optimal functioning of organs and tissues is promoted, influencing holistic health, both physically and emotionally. This is a comprehensive discipline that addresses health and well-being holistically, recognizing the importance of nutrition, emotional balance, and maintenance of physical health. Therefore, it is essential to nourish ourselves properly, consuming foods that satisfy our needs and cover all tastes. Additionally, it is important to consider our dosha when selecting our foods, as this can significantly contribute to our overall health.

Knowing which foods are harmful and beneficial for our dosha can significantly improve our well-being.

AYURVEDA TEST

By taking this test, we determine the percentage of the three Dosha spheres: Vata, Pitta, and Kapha, and determine your Ayurvedic constitution.

Take your time to select according to each characteristic the one that best fits you.

PHYSICAL STRUCTURE

1. **Body Build**

v) Thin, small.

p) Medium.

k) Large, heavy, strong.

2. **Weight**

v) Thin, difficulty gaining weight.

p) Medium, maintains a stable weight.

k) Generally overweight, easily gains weight.

3. **Complexion**

v) Brown, tan.

p) Fair, reddish or yellowish tint.

k) Pale, porcelain-like.

4. **Skin**

v) Thin, rough, cold; dry skin and dark tone.

p) Soft, warm, prone to acne, moles, and freckles, easily burns in the sun, reddish.

k) Smooth, soft, thick, clear, shiny, late appearance of wrinkles.

5. Hair

v) Dry, thin, brittle, wavy.

p) Greasy, straight, with gray hair or early baldness.

k) Thick, strong, wavy or curly, oily.

6. Face

v) Oval.

p) Pointed/well-defined jawline.

k) Round.

7. Forehead

v) Small.

p) Medium.

k) Large.

8. Eyes

v) Small, dry, dull.

p) Medium, prone to redness, intense, sharp.

k) Large, round, bright, relaxed, moist.

9. Nose

v) Uneven shape, deviated septum.

p) Long, pointed nose tip, often red.

k) Button nose, short, rounded.

10. Teeth

v) Large, crooked, spaced, thin gums.

p) Medium size, yellowish, soft gums.

k) White, strong, even, strong gums.

11. Hands

v) Dry, rough, thin fingers.

p) Moist, warm or pink, medium fingers.

k) Firm, thick hand, thick fingers.

12. **Nails**

v) Dry, rough, brittle.

p) Soft, flexible, pink.

k) Strong, thick, smooth.

13. **Chest**

v) Small, flat, sunken.

p) Medium size.

k) Large, wide, expanded.

14. **Joints**

v) Small, prominent bones.

p) Medium size.

k) Large, sturdy, lubricated.

15. **Veins and Tendons**

v) Prominent, noticeable.

p) Loose tendons and ligaments.

k) Well-covered.

PHYSIOLOGICAL CHARACTERISTICS

16. Sweating

v) Hardly sweats during any activity.

p) Sweats profusely even with minimal activity.

k) Minimal sweating during moderate activity or in summer.

17. Thirst

v) Variable.

p) Strong.

k) Low.

18. Appetite

v) Variable appetite, anxious when hungry.

p) Strong, cannot skip meals, might get angry, irritable when hungry.

k) Stable, regular, can go without eating.

19. Digestion

v) Irregular.

p) Fast.

k) Slow.

20. Indigestion leads to:

v) Constipation, gas, bloating.

p) Heartburn, acid reflux.

k) Mucus.

21. Bowel Movement

v) Dry, often constipated.

p) Loose, often 2-3 times a day.

k) Loose, slow, once a day.

22. Preferred Tastes

v) Sweet, salty, sour.

p) Sweet, bitter, astringent.

k) Bitter, spicy, astringent.

23. Preferred Climate

v) Warm, humid.

p) Cold and dry.

k) Warm and dry. Can tolerate extremes.

24. Voice

v) Weak, hoarse.

p) Strong and loud.

k) Deep, melodious.

25. Speech

v) Rapid, scattered speech, talkative, easily diverted from the topic.

p) Fast, clear, precise speech, very good communicator.

k) Slow, clear, quiet, monotone.

26. Endurance

v) Low.

p) Moderate.

k) High.

27. Sleep Pattern

v) Short and interrupted.

p) Moderate, can fall back asleep if wakes up at night.

k) Long, deep, can easily sleep for 8 to 10 hours.

28. Dreams

v) Multiple, rapid, fearful. Often sees wind and air.

p) Fiery, often conflicting. Often sees fire.

k) Romantic, slow, happy. Often sees water.

BEHAVIORAL CHARACTERISTICS

29. Nature/Temperament

v) Anxious, nervous. Worries too much.

p) Often irritable and angry. Gets nervous.

k) Relaxed, caring, affectionate.

30. Actions

v) Quick and spontaneous.

p) Very precise and organized.

k) Slow and graceful.

31. Activities

v) Very active. Multitasking.

p) Planned and calculated activities.

k) Slow and steady. Cannot multitask.

32. Courage

v) Easily frightened.

p) Very brave.

k) Moderate.

33. Mind

v) Constant thoughts, restless.

p) Impatient.

k) Calm, peaceful.

34. This phrase defines me

v) I like to learn about everything, but I don't delve deep.

p) It doesn't matter how, just get it done.

k) I prefer to conserve my energy.

35. Faith or beliefs

v) Variable.

p) Strong dedication.

k) Consistent.

36. Intellectual Response

v) Quick, not detailed.

p) Precise and timely competence.

k) With rhythm, but accurate.

37. Memory

v) Good short-term memory. Quick to forget.

p) Average but precise.

k) With rhythm, but accurate.

38. **Shopping Style**

v) Impulse buyer.

p) Brand-conscious.

k) Money saver.

39. **Relationships**

v) Flexible and easily adapts to different people.

p) Passionate.

k) Rigid, fixed, not adaptable.

40. **Friendships**

v) Short-term. Several friends.

p) Chooses friends based on values and merits.

k) Slow to make new friends, very loyal.

41. **Interests and Hobbies**

v) Anything related to movement and expansion like art, dance, and travel.

p) Anything related to status, intense feelings like sports, politics.

k) Enjoys tranquility and not exceeding or spending energy.

42. If you had to describe yourself, which word applies most to you?

v) Nomad.

p) Leader.

k) Carefree.

43. I like

v) Creativity, the artistic, moving all the time: dance, travel.

p) Intense passion: sports, politics.

k) Quiet and relaxing activities: knitting, pottery, reading books, poetry.

44. **The motto of my life is**

v) Expressing myself, art, creativity, dance.

p) Leaving my mark on the world and being famous.

k) Helping, supporting, and nurturing others.

SCORE: Please count each response you selected with V), P), and K), and place them in each box.

VATA: _________________

PITTA: _________________

KAPHA: _________________

According to your highest score, your Dosha constitution is:

Characteristics of Vata Dosha:

VATA

***Combination of ether and air**: Associated with mobility, dryness, lightness, and coldness. People with this predominance are usually creative, energetic, inconsistent, ingenious, and may experience rapid mood changes.

***Digestion**: Variable digestion, tendency towards irregularity, and sensitivity to certain foods.

***Bone structure**: Thin bones and prominent joints, making them more prone to stiffness and joint discomfort.

***Temperament**: Associated with creativity, inconsistency, and versatility. People with a predominance of Vata are usually emotionally sensitive and creative but may also experience anxiety and worry.

Pitta:

***Combination of fire and water**. It is associated with digestion, metabolism, heat, and intensity. People with this predominance are ambitious, energetic, problem-solvers, strong-tempered, and have good leadership skills.

***Digestion**: People with a predominance of Pitta tend to have strong and quick digestion, often experiencing heartburn and sensitivity to spicy or fatty foods.

***Bone Structure**: They tend to have a medium bone structure and well-defined musculature, which can make them more prone to inflammation and excess acidity in the body.

***Temperament**: The Pitta temperament is associated with intensity, passion, and determination. People with this predominance are usually energetic, ambitious, and strong-tempered, but they can also be prone to getting angry easily.

Kapha:

***Combination of water and earth.**

It is associated with stability, solidity, calmness, and freshness.

People with a predominance of Kapha tend to be loving, compassionate, patient, calm, and have good physical endurance.

***Digestion**: People with a predominance of Kapha tend to have stable and slow digestion, but they may be prone to mucus buildup and slow digestion.

***Bone Structure**: They have a solid bone structure and well-developed musculature, which provides them with stability and endurance, but they may also be prone to fluid retention.

***Temperament**: The Kapha temperament is associated with stability, calmness, and compassion. People with this predominance are usually loving, patient, and have a calm nature, but they may also experience stubbornness and resistance to change.

Drinks for Each Dosha.

Each dosha has unique properties to balance each one through appropriate food and beverages. Here are some beverages; there are many more, and it is recommended to adjust them for each case and particular preferences.

Vata

Drinks for Vata Dosha:

Ginger tea: Mix hot water with fresh ginger slices and let it steep for a few minutes before drinking. Ginger helps stimulate digestion and soothe Vata imbalances.

Fennel infusion: Boil fennel seeds in water for a few minutes. Fennel is beneficial for relieving bloating and gas, common issues in Vata imbalances. Other recommended drinks include cinnamon tea, clove tea, aloe vera juice, apple juice, cherry juice, grape juice, mango juice, among others.

PITTA

Drinks for Pitta Dosha:

Rosewater: Add a few drops of rosewater to a glass of fresh water. Rosewater has refreshing properties and helps balance the heat and acidity associated with Pitta.

Coriander infusion: Boil coriander seeds in water for a few minutes. Coriander has refreshing properties and can help alleviate stomach acidity and irritation related to Pitta.

KAPHA

Drinks for Kapha Dosha:

Ginger and lemon tea: Mix hot water with slices of fresh ginger and a few drops of lemon juice. Ginger helps stimulate digestion, while lemon adds a refreshing and acidic flavor to balance Kapha.

Cinnamon infusion: Boil a cinnamon stick in water for a few minutes. Cinnamon has stimulating properties and helps balance Kapha imbalances, improving digestion

"Remember, all illnesses have a specific trigger of feelings, emotions, and dietary disorder"

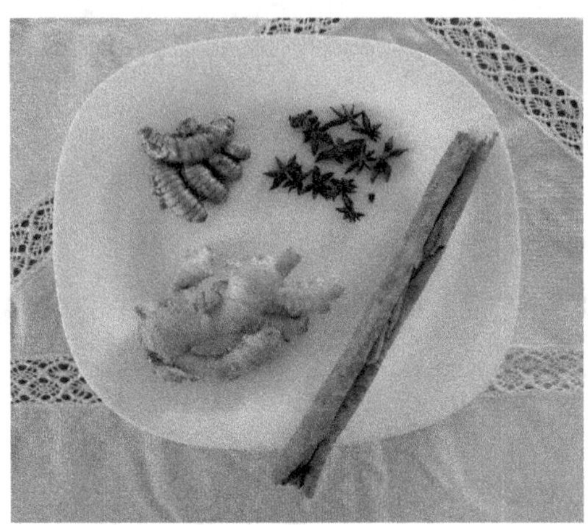

"If you have noticed that you have a predominantly Vata constitution, it is crucial to make adjustments in your lifestyle to balance this Dosha. As a Vata person, I have experienced these challenges and have sought ways to balance myself. Here are some general recommendations that have been very helpful for me:

1. Establish a daily routine that includes moments for meditation, rest, and relaxation. Consistency and calmness are essential to soothe Vata.

2. Maintain regular meal times and ensure that they are warm, nutritious, and comforting. Simple and fresh food can help counteract Vata's restless nature.

3. Avoid excessive activity and aim to reserve moments of tranquility. Rest and pause are essential to counteract the tendency toward excess movement and mental activity.

4. Incorporate foods and flavors that are comforting and nutritious, such as stews, soups, and foods rich in oil and healthy fats. These can provide stability and warmth to the Vata body.

5. Seek gentle activities and exercises that help you stay grounded and connected to your body, such as gentle yoga, tai chi, or quiet walks in nature. Gentle and mindful movement can counteract the tendency toward dispersion and instability.

When Vata is in balance, it fosters creativity, flexibility, and evokes feelings of freshness, lightness, happiness, and joy. Out of balance, Vata produces fear, nervousness, anxiety, even tremors and spasms. Vata is dry, light, cold, subtle, clear, mobile, and scattered.

Remember that these recommendations are based on my personal experience as a Vata person. If possible, I would recommend seeking the advice of an Ayurvedic professional for a more specific and personalized plan.

The great sage physician Charaka, one of the founders of Ayurvedic medicine, said: 'A physician, though well versed in the knowledge and treatment of disease, who does not enter the patient's heart with the virtue of light and love, will not be able to cure the patient.' If only all health workers followed this wise advice.

The whole journey of life is divided into three main milestones. From birth to 16 years old is the Kapha age. From 16 to 50 is the Pitta age, and from 50 to 100 is the Vata age. When it is not possible to be in harmony and balance from an early age, these milestones are not fulfilled; we must help our body and mind in a simple and permanent way so that you can lead a healthy life.

'Feed your body with warmth, stability, and love; it is feeding the soul. Every bite is an opportunity to nourish internal balance, strengthening our being on all levels'".

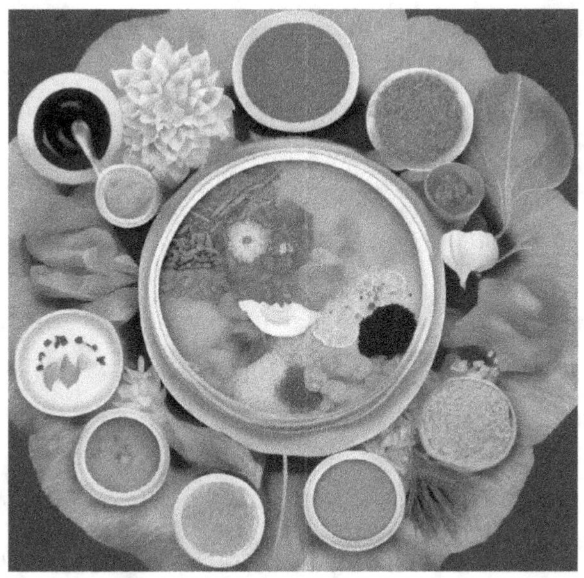

Chapter 2

What privileges do you have when practicing meditation?

"Meditation is the food of the spirit,

the calm of the mind"

Meditation is a practice that involves training the mind to achieve a state of focused attention, mental clarity, and relaxation. Often associated with spiritual and religious traditions, it has also become popular as a tool for overall mental and emotional well-being.

43

The benefits of meditation are diverse and include stress and anxiety reduction, increased concentration and attention, fostering creativity, developing compassion and empathy, promoting self-awareness, and spiritual connection, among others.

This is a versatile practice that can contribute to improving people's well-being and quality of life in various aspects.

It fosters greater compassion towards others. Compassion involves feeling empathy when witnessing the suffering of others and urges us to help alleviate their pain. Unlike empathy, compassion includes the willingness to end the suffering of others, leading us to act compassionately in various situations, such as accompanying someone sick in the hospital, helping those with learning difficulties, or providing financial support to those in need.

The practice of meditation helps you acquire wisdom to know and identify your physical, mental, and energetic body. As you immerse yourself in it, you begin to connect more consciously with your body, identifying each part and developing motor skills, balance, and confidence to maintain a healthy lifestyle.

Meditation allows you to become acquainted with the sources of happiness, those pleasant moments stored in your memory with love. This self-awareness helps improve your mood and allows you to let thoughts flow freely, like birds in the sky.

It is crucial that the posture you adopt during meditation allows you to be relaxed and comfortable while keeping you alert and aware. This way, you can fully enjoy your meditation session and release underlying physical and emotional tensions. A natural spine alignment, relaxed shoulders, and balance of the head and face are key aspects of proper posture.

Each meditation posture has its own advantages and challenges, and the choice of posture will depend on the comfort and physical capacity of each individual. The lotus posture and half-lotus posture are the most traditional, but it is important to find a posture that allows you to maintain comfort and concentration during meditation practice. Here are some of them.

- **Sitting on a chair**: Position your buttocks slightly higher than your knees by tilting your pelvis forward, keeping your back straight and your shoulders relaxed. Using a small cushion can provide greater comfort.

Let the energy of the surrounding nature flow through you, feel how the fresh air nourishes your being. Let the presence of the trees remind you to grow and reach your full potential while remaining firmly rooted in the present moment.

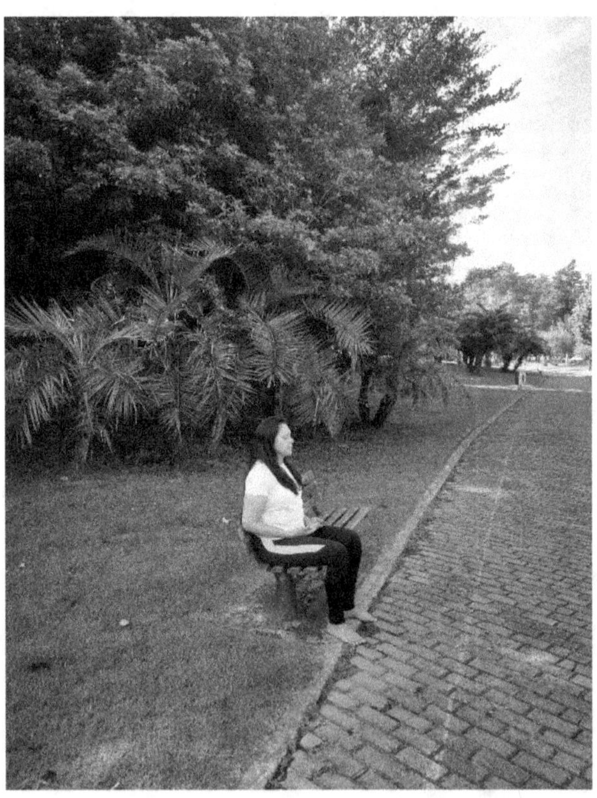

47

- **Walking meditation**: As the Zen master says, "walk as if you are kissing the earth with your feet". Keep your back upright and relaxed, with your shoulders loose, and direct your head towards the sky. Feel the weight of your feet in contact with the earth or the ground with each step, preferably barefoot and unhurried, presently in the here and now.

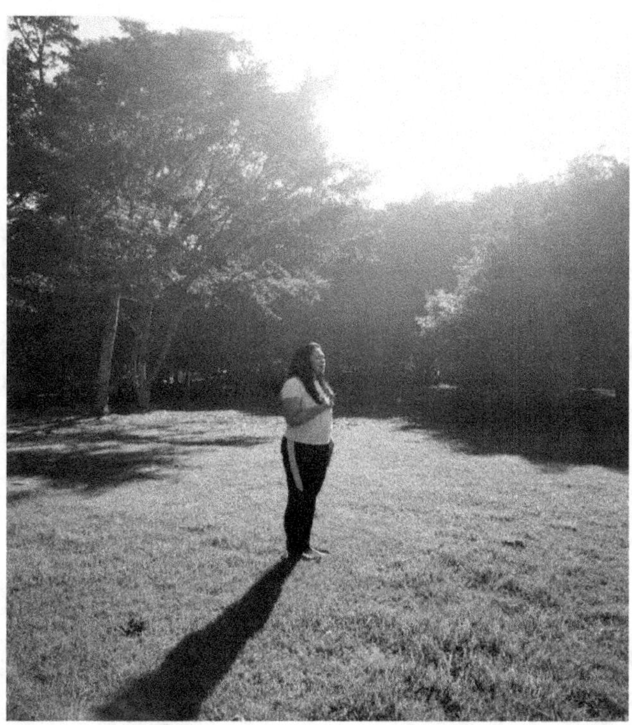

- **Lotus posture with supports**: The thighs should rest on a yoga block and the knees should be directed towards the ground. If the knees do not touch the ground, it is important to use a blanket or blocks to avoid pinching the internal meniscus. This posture is more comfortable on the ground and allows for an intermediate height.

In the spiritual practices of various traditions, importance is given to the lotus position as a posture that facilitates energy flow and aids in the search for enlightenment or mental clarity.

By using support such as cushions, yoga blocks, or blankets, the practitioner can adjust the position to be as comfortable as possible, thus facilitating a longer and more fruitful practice of meditation or pranayama. It is important to note that each individual is different and should adapt practices like yoga to their unique needs and abilities.

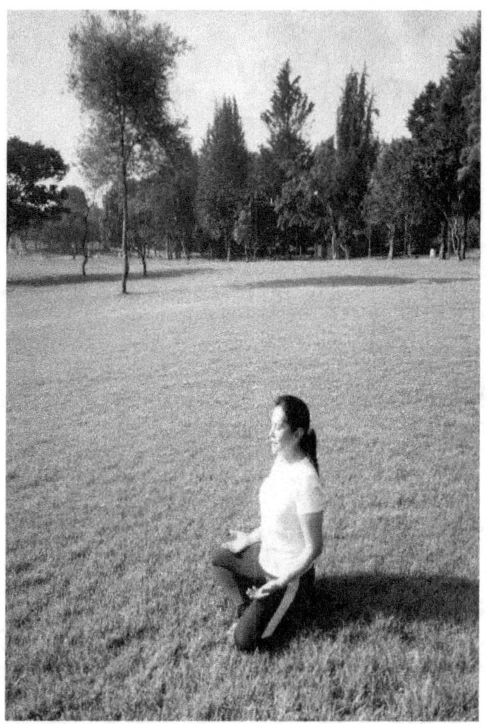

The kneeling meditation posture is often referred to as virasana. To do this posture, you should:

- Kneel on the floor with your knees together and your toes separated, so that the buttocks rest between the heels.

- If your buttocks do not reach the heels, you can place a cushion or a folded blanket between the heels and the buttocks for greater comfort.

- Keep the spine straight and the shoulders relaxed. You can place your hands on your knees or in your lap.

- Breathe gently and relax your body, allowing your attention to focus on meditation.

It is important to remember that if you feel any pain or discomfort in your knees or ankles while doing this posture, it is advisable to consult a yoga instructor for additional guidance.

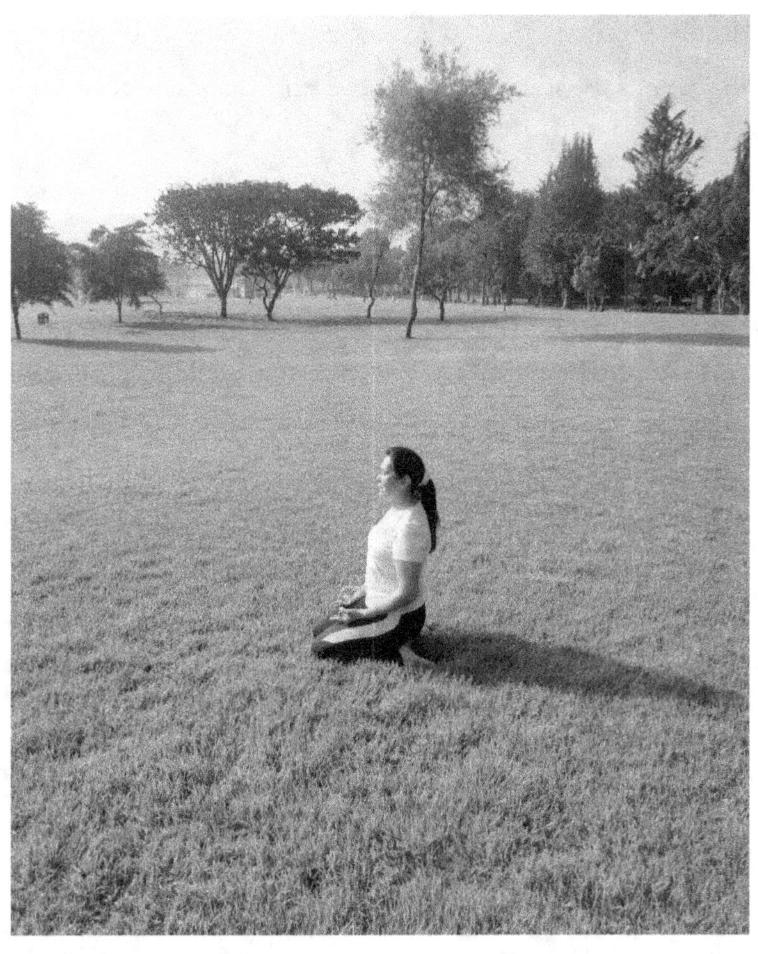

- Lying down: This posture requires more attention and concentration to focus awareness on the breath. Although it is easy to associate the lying position with sleeping, meditating is the opposite of sleeping: it is a state of wakeful mindfulness and concentration. Stay relaxed, but not asleep. Experiment with various postures and choose the one that feels most comfortable.

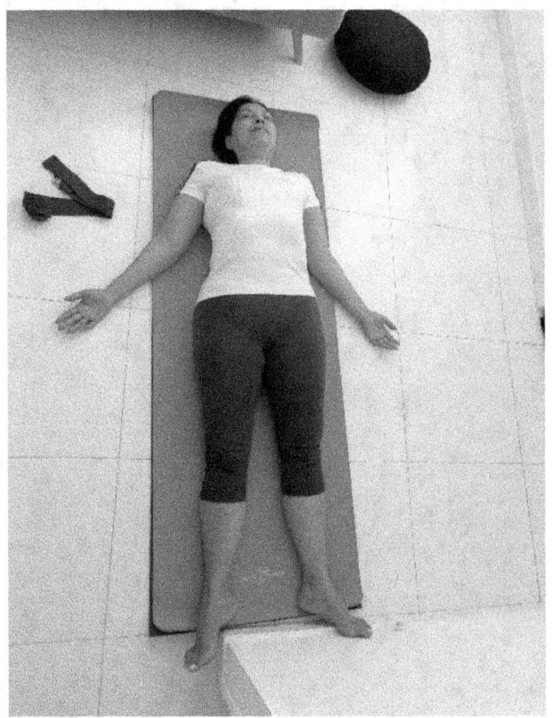

Breathing: Since the brain needs to focus on something, focusing on the breath is an excellent way to clear the mind. You should sit in your favorite meditation position and start focusing all your attention on the rhythm of your breath, the sound it makes as it enters and exits through the nose, and the sensation of the air as it does so.

Conscious Breathing.

Conscious breathing is a practice that involves focusing attention on the act of breathing, being fully aware of each inhalation and exhalation. This technique is not only central to meditation and yoga practices but is also used in relaxation therapies and stress reduction programs.

Principles of conscious breathing:

- **Mindfulness**: Complete attention is paid to the breath, feeling how the air enters and exits the body.

- **Natural Rhythm**: The rhythm of breathing is not attempted to be controlled but observed and allowed to find its own natural rhythm.

- **Body-Mind Connection**: Through observing the breath, a greater connection between the body and mind can be achieved, bringing a state of serenity.

- **Awareness of the Present Moment**: Concentrating on the breath helps anchor the mind in the present moment, reducing the propensity to be distracted by thoughts about the past or worries about the future.

How to practice conscious breathing:

1. Find a comfortable and quiet place to sit or lie down.

2. Close your eyes to reduce visual distractions and focus internally.

3. Begin to observe your natural breathing, without trying to change it.

4. Notice how the air fills your lungs and how your abdomen rises and falls with each breath.

5. If your mind starts to wander, gently redirect it back to your breath.

6. Practice for a set time or until you feel calmer and more centered.

This practice can be performed by almost anyone, regardless of age or physical condition, and can be a powerful tool for improving quality of life and overall well-being.

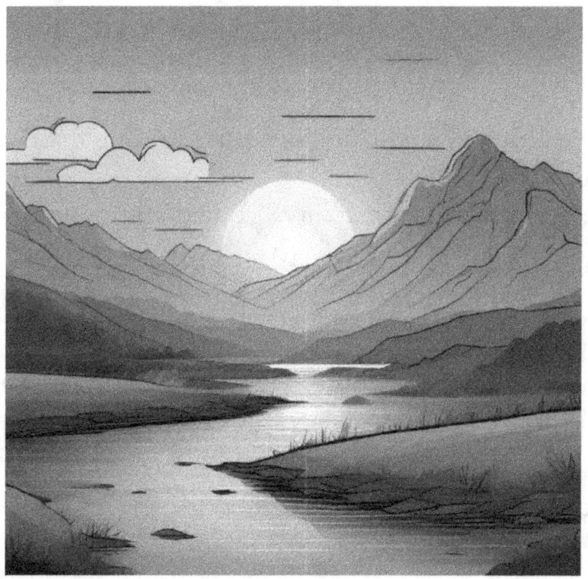

When you can be in a place like this: You should breathe deeply and feel the water in the mountains, it is an act of generosity towards our body and mind.

Chapter 3

Yoga

> "Listening to music or practicing art are activities
>
> that nourish both the mind and the spirit"

Yoga is an ancient practice with a wide range of benefits, both for the mind and the body. It combines postures with conscious breathing, leading to a series of tangible health and well-being benefits. Among them are:

1. Improved flexibility: Practicing yoga regularly increases flexibility by stretching muscles, tendons, and ligaments. Over time, postures that initially seem impossible can become more accessible.

2. Muscle strengthening: Many yoga postures are designed to strengthen different muscle groups. Better muscle tone not only improves physical appearance but also protects against conditions like arthritis and relieves back pain.

3. Improved posture: Yoga practice promotes body awareness, which helps in developing better and more upright posture. Yoga postures not only strengthen the body but also empower the mind. By practicing yoga, a sense of inner strength is fostered, and fear of making decisions is reduced.

This discipline helps block out external noise and connect solely with one's internal self, leading to greater self-confidence.

4. Increased blood circulation: Exercise in yoga promotes circulation, especially in the limbs, which can help reduce inflammation and increase hemoglobin and red blood cell levels.

It also improves blood pressure and heart rate: Studies have shown that "yoga can reduce resting blood pressure and heart rate, contributing to improved long-term cardiovascular risk" (source: Canadian Journal of Cardiology). This discipline goes beyond stretching muscles as it positively impacts heart health and the circulatory system in general.

5. Provides an energy boost: Many individuals report feeling more energized and revitalized after a yoga session, as the practice stimulates various bodily systems such as digestion, circulation, and the nervous system.

6. Stress reduction: Yoga is known for its ability to relax the mind and reduce stress levels through breathing techniques (pranayama), meditation, and conscious posture execution.

7. Improves concentration: Regular yoga practice enhances concentration, coordination, memory, and even intellectual quotient.

Yoga practice requires full attention and concentration on the present moment, which contributes to greater mental clarity and physical coordination. Learning to maintain concentration during yoga postures can foster a greater ability to focus on various daily tasks.

8. Regulation of adrenaline and cortisol: Yoga can reduce cortisol levels, a hormone released in response to stress. Elevated cortisol levels can influence blood pressure, immune system suppression, and obesity. Stress and anxiety reduction: Yoga promotes relaxation by reducing cortisol and cholesterol levels in the blood through relaxation movements that help balance the nervous system. Regular yoga practice can help counteract negative thoughts and promote a calmer and more balanced mental state.

9. Improves sleep quality: By reducing stress and promoting relaxation, yoga can improve sleep quality.

10. Mental health benefits: Yoga is effective in improving mental health, addressing conditions such as

depression, anxiety, post-traumatic stress disorder (PTSD), and insomnia.

11. Improves digestion: Yoga movements can stimulate the digestive system, helping to alleviate digestive problems. Many yoga postures involve gentle and fluid movements that can stimulate the digestive tract and contribute to better digestion. Forward bends and twists, for example, can exert gentle pressure on the intestines, promoting the elimination of feces and gases. This practice can be beneficial for those seeking to support their digestive health.

One yoga posture that is considered beneficial for the digestive system is the seated spinal twist. To perform it, sit on the floor with your legs extended. Then, bend your right knee and place the right foot next to the left knee. Bring the left arm around the right knee and twist to the right, placing the right hand on the floor behind you for support. Hold the posture for several deep breaths and then repeat on the other side.

This posture helps stimulate the digestive system and alleviates abdominal discomfort. It's always important to consult with a professional before attempting new exercises, especially if you have pre-existing medical conditions.

12. Immune system stimulation: Yoga aids in stimulating the lymphatic system, which plays a vital role in fighting infections and removing toxins from the body.

These benefits accrue with regular practice and contribute to overall well-being. However, it's important to note that benefits may vary from person to person, and it's always recommended to practice under the guidance of a qualified instructor, especially for beginners or those with specific health conditions.

We can say that meditation and yoga are two complementary practices that offer significant benefits for both the body and mind, allowing for a comprehensive approach to a higher quality of life.

Whenever you perform postures, invite your body to accept all of them, with the intention of relieving, strengthening, and healing whatever is bothering you in your body and mind; it's also a way to become aware and encourage ourselves to do them with joy and enthusiasm.

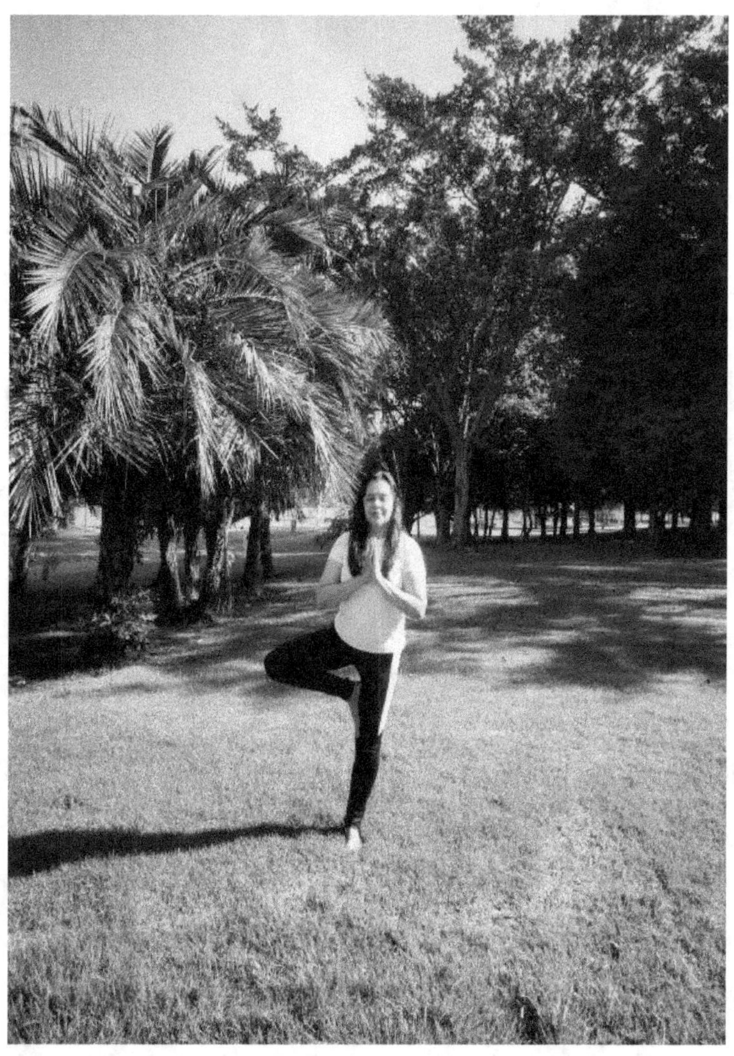

Chapter 4

Inner Child

"Laughter is a balm for the body

and the best elixir for the mind"

The "inner child" represents the part of us that retains the experiences, emotions, and memories of childhood. This aspect of our psyche can influence our adult lives in significant ways. The inner child can manifest through our emotional responses, behavior patterns, and deeply rooted beliefs, many of which originate from our interactions and experiences during childhood.

Connecting with our inner child provides us with the opportunity to explore and heal existing emotional wounds, address limiting beliefs, and reconnect with the innocence, joy, and creativity that characterize childhood. By becoming aware of our inner child, we can take steps to care for and nurture this part of ourselves, thereby facilitating more complete personal and emotional growth.

It is essential to understand that the inner child does not simply represent the chronological age of childhood but rather the experiences and emotions that have left a lasting imprint on our psyche. By embracing and understanding our inner child, we can foster self-acceptance, compassion, and emotional healing on the path to a more fulfilling and satisfying life.

Psychology, especially through psychoanalysis, has highlighted the importance of childhood in our development as adults. Therapy aimed at healing emotional wounds and traumas from childhood can help connect with the inherent love and joy we experienced upon entering the world, thereby transforming pain into maturity and preventing it from becoming suffering. This emotional healing provides us with the opportunity to discover our true power and promote positive change in our lives as we overcome fears and deprogram harmful patterns.

Each of us is composed of three parts: the parent, the adult, and the inner child. These three parts influence our perception of the world, our relationships, and our personal growth. It is essential to recognize and understand how our childhood experiences have shaped our identity and behavior.

Within these parts exist different ego states that can manifest positively or negatively. For example, the "Parent" represents our norms and beliefs, the "Adult" carries out practical and efficient actions, while the "Child" harbors our emotional needs and our creativity and imagination.

To achieve a healthy balance, it is necessary to harmoniously integrate these three parts of our psyche. The "Parent" must be demanding and compassionate, the "Adult" must carry out necessary actions, and the "Child" must receive the attention and emotional care it needs.

If you feel stuck in your life, have difficulties in your personal and work relationships, face emotional or physical challenges, or experience stress, anxiety, or depression, you may need to release beliefs and memories from the past and reestablish a relationship with your inner child. By providing your inner child with the attention and care it needs, you can find emotional relief and promote greater balance and satisfaction in your life.

Healing Our Inner Child: A Journey of Self-Discovery and Personal Growth

Therapy aimed at healing emotional wounds and traumas from childhood can help us reconnect with our authentic essence, promoting transformative change that allows us to live more meaningfully and fully.

Remembrance and Reconstruction:

- Remember and reconstruct childhood memories, identifying your favorite programs and activities that you enjoyed. This process will help you remember who you were and where you longed to go in your childhood.

Forgiveness and Release:

- Healing emotional wounds from the past requires learning to forgive and release old resentments. This can illuminate your vision for the future and provide clarity in the present.

Reclaiming Dreams and Joys:

- Identify and pursue those dreams you once abandoned. What did you want to do as a child? Embrace the opportunity to reclaim those desires and bring them back to life; it's never too late to honor your passions.

Reclaiming Fun and Wonder:

- Affirm your capacity for wonder and enjoy simple and wonderful moments. Allow yourself to play, enjoy innocence, and be carried away by fun.

Important Connections:

- Strengthen your bonds and emotional relationships; allow your parents or significant figures in your life to nurture and protect you. This emotional connection can provide comfort and support on your healing journey.

Spontaneity and Creativity:

- Find moments of spontaneity and creativity in your daily life. Allow yourself to experiment with new activities and rediscover the freedom that comes with genuine expression of the inner self.

Reconnect with Childhood Happiness:

- Free yourself from daily pressures and enjoy moments of childlike fun. Let the satisfaction and joy of feeling like a child return to your life, even for a day.

Self-Love and Protection:

- Learn to unconditionally love your inner child, offering protection, care, and love. Allowing it to express itself freely can become the source of lasting joy and happiness.

It is important to remember that emotional experiences from childhood, both positive and negative, can shape our perceptions and beliefs throughout life. Healing our inner child provides us with the opportunity to free ourselves from past emotional burdens and promote significant personal growth.

By embracing our inner child with compassion and care, we can open ourselves to a more fulfilling and meaningful life. Remember that each of these actions can contribute to deep emotional healing and greater well-being in the present.

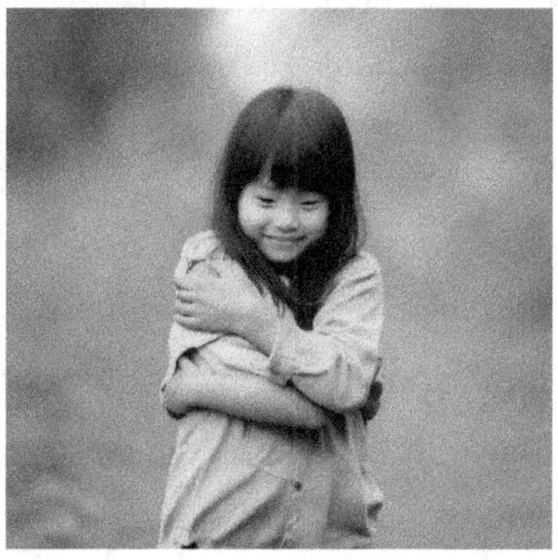

Chapter 5

Biological Decoding

> "Self-care is an act of self-love
>
> that nurtures both body anmind"

Biological decoding is a therapeutic approach based on the concept that the physical and emotional symptoms we experience are manifestations of the body's adaptation process to emotional stress or inner conflicts. This approach considers the connection between the body, mind, and emotions, seeking to understand the biological and emotional origins of diseases and physical symptoms.

Practitioners of biological decoding believe that physical symptoms are the body's attempt to resolve unresolved emotional conflicts and seek to identify and address the underlying emotions and beliefs that may be contributing to the manifestation of the illness.

Through biological decoding, the goal is to identify each individual's "personal history," understanding their emotional experiences, internal conflicts, and traumatic experiences, with the purpose of finding connections between these aspects and the physical symptoms they may be experiencing. The ultimate objective is to address these emotional conflicts comprehensively, through emotional understanding and expression, therapy, and, in some cases, lifestyle changes.

Biological decoding therapy also provides a tool for promoting conscious and full health by addressing past emotions and experiences that impact how we relate to ourselves and others. This therapeutic approach focuses on helping individuals understand and overcome various emotional issues such as depression, anxiety, post-traumatic stress, and trauma-related disorders.

It is crucial to recognize that our past experiences, both positive and negative, leave a mark on our minds and bodies. Beliefs and emotions rooted in childhood, adolescence, and even ancestral history have a significant impact on how we relate to the world, others, and ourselves. Decoding therapy seeks to unravel these connections and provide a space for emotional healing.

Furthermore, it is essential to reflect on the power of our words and thoughts. Our personal history and the words that have defined us over the years have a powerful effect on our perception of ourselves and the world around us.

Understanding this gives us the opportunity to undergo deep healing through love and self-discovery.

Decoding therapy has the potential to unlock repressed emotions, change unwanted behavioral patterns, and promote a greater sense of self-confidence and well-being. By learning to honor our life stories, we can pave the way for healing and personal growth.

Remember that biological decoding therapy requires commitment and loyalty to oneself for effective and lasting healing; otherwise, confusion may arise, and one may think it is not yielding good results. Maintaining a space for emotional and spiritual healing is essential for addressing life's challenges with understanding and love, and to support the overall well-being of each individual.

It is important to note that biological decoding is a complementary therapeutic approach and does not replace conventional medical treatments. If you are considering biological decoding as a therapeutic method, I would recommend seeking out a certified professional and discussing your decision with a trusted doctor or therapist.

"I would like to share some steps that a therapist can follow when practicing Biological Decoding to address depression. Personally, I found

that studying this discipline helped me identify signals that my body was transmitting through pain, which was very helpful for my healing process".

- Personal History: The therapist examines the patient's personal history, including traumatic events, relationships, losses, and other stress factors that may have contributed to their current state.

- Seeking Emotional Conflict: The attempt is made to identify the emotional conflict that, according to the theory of biological decoding, is manifesting the depression. For example, one could interpret that depression is linked to a symbolic loss or a conflict of identity or self-worth within the individual's life story.

- Mind-Body Connection: Emphasis is placed on the connection between emotions and physiology, seeking how the body may be "expressing" what the mind has not been able to resolve.

- Therapeutic Technique: Through techniques such as dialogue, visualization, or relaxation techniques, the aim is to unlock the emotional conflict found and allow for a healthy expression and processing of those emotions.

- Follow-up and Support: Ongoing support is provided to help the patient integrate any new understanding or emotional change and ensure they can handle any emotion or memory that may have arisen during therapy.

It is important to note that biological decoding is not widely recognized or practiced in conventional clinical settings. Evidence of its effectiveness is anecdotal and not supported by mainstream scientific research to the extent that other psychological treatments for depression, such as cognitive-behavioral therapy or pharmacological treatments, are.

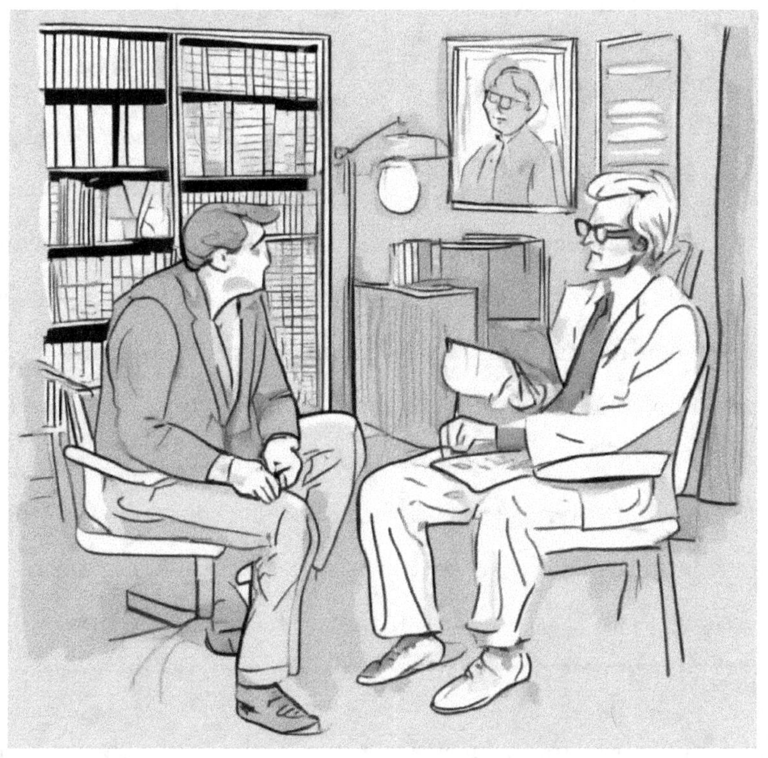

Chapter 6

Orthomolecular Nutrition

> "Speaking kindly to oneself is crucial
>
> for maintaining a healthy mind"

Orthomolecular nutrition is an alternative medicine approach that focuses on using nutrients in therapeutic doses to prevent and treat diseases. The term "orthomolecular" was coined by chemist Linus Pauling in the 1960s and derives from "ortho," which means correct or appropriate. The fundamental premise of orthomolecular nutrition is that providing the body with the correct amounts of essential nutrients can restore biochemical balance and promote optimal health.

In orthomolecular nutrition, many diseases are considered to result from nutritional imbalances or deficiencies of vitamins, minerals, amino acids, and essential fatty acids. Therefore, treatment focuses on identifying these deficiencies and correcting them through dietary supplementation.

Key nutrients used in orthomolecular nutrition include vitamin C, vitamin D, B vitamins, omega-3 fatty acids, magnesium, zinc, and antioxidants. These nutrients are administered in individualized doses, usually under the supervision of a healthcare professional trained in orthomolecular medicine.

The benefits of orthomolecular nutrition are evident in supporting various health conditions, from common colds to more serious diseases such as cancer. For example, vitamin C has been shown to be effective for both the common cold and in treating terminal cancer patients. Additionally, research has revealed that vitamin B3 may contribute to reducing anxiety, treating addictions, and benefiting patients with schizophrenia by addressing nutritional deficiencies in the brain.

Furthermore, orthomolecular nutrition addresses a wide range of diseases, including cardiovascular diseases, diabetes, obesity, hypothyroidism, cancer, kidney stones, and circulation problems. This form of nutrition has been observed to offer positive outcomes in 90% of conditions.

Lastly, the use of nutrients such as zinc has been shown to be effective in preventing viral replication and protecting cell membranes, which can be beneficial in treating various diseases.

Orthomolecular nutrition in renal patients must be handled with extreme care, as their kidneys have reduced capacity to filter and eliminate excess nutrients such as potassium, phosphorus, and sodium. We must consider some points:

1. Electrolyte Control: Patients with kidney disease often need to control their intake of electrolytes such as potassium, phosphorus, and sodium, as their accumulation can be dangerous. Supplementation should be carefully monitored to avoid imbalances.

2. Proteins: The amount of protein needed may vary. Some patients may need to limit their protein intake to reduce the burden on the kidneys, while others, at different stages of kidney disease or on dialysis, may need more protein. Protein quality is also crucial.

3. Fluid Control: Managing fluid intake is critical in patients with advanced kidney disease to avoid fluid overload, which can lead to complications such as hypertension and heart failure.

4. Vitamins and Minerals: Deficiency of certain vitamins and minerals is common in kidney disease, but supplementation should be done cautiously, avoiding

overdoses, especially of those nutrients that are eliminated through the kidneys.

5. Phosphorus Control: Phosphorus intake should be closely monitored because elevated phosphorus levels can contribute to bone diseases in patients with kidney disease.

6. Regular Visits to the Nutritionist: Regular follow-up with a nutritionist, preferably one specialized in renal management, is essential to adjust the nutritional plan as the patient's needs change and to avoid any adverse effects.

7. Caution with Supplements: Many supplements contain high levels of minerals or ingredients that may be harmful to people with reduced kidney function. A healthcare professional should always be consulted before starting any new supplementation.

Orthomolecular nutrition may have potential benefits for patients with renal deficiency; it must be administered with careful planning and constant professional supervision to ensure that it positively contributes to the patient's health without causing additional complications.

Orthomolecular nutrition recommends a diet rich in:

- Fruits and vegetables: These foods are rich in vitamins, minerals, antioxidants, and fiber.

- Whole grains: Whole grains provide fiber, B vitamins, and minerals.

- Lean proteins: Lean proteins, such as chicken, fish, and beans, are essential for muscle health, immune function, and tissue repair.

- Healthy fats: Healthy fats, such as those found in avocado, olive oil, and nuts, are important for heart health, brain function, and hormone regulation.

Orthomolecular nutrition also recommends avoiding or limiting the following foods:

* Processed foods: Processed foods are often high in sugar, unhealthy fats, and sodium, which can contribute to health problems.

* Refined sugar: Refined sugar can cause inflammation, weight gain, and dental caries.

*   Trans fats: Trans fats are artificial fats that have been linked to heart disease and other health issues.

*   Fried foods: Fried foods are often high in unhealthy fats and can increase the risk of chronic diseases.

Here are some specific examples of foods recommended by orthomolecular nutrition:

- Fruits: Berries, citrus fruits, apples, bananas

- Vegetables: Broccoli, kale, spinach, carrots, tomatoes

- Whole grains: Brown rice, quinoa, oats, whole wheat bread

- Lean proteins: Chicken, fish, tofu, beans, lentils

- Healthy fats: Avocado, olive oil, nuts, seeds, etc.

Chapter 7

Activation of the Pineal Gland

"Connection with nature

is medicine for the body and soul"

The activation of the pineal gland is a process that can be guided by an experienced professional and is often associated with emotional well-being and quality of life. In exploring this journey, it is crucial to understand that the pineal gland, located at the center of the brain, plays a significant role in the secretion of melatonin, directly impacting the quality of sleep.

Philosophy, psychology, and biology teach us that self-awareness is fundamental. It's not about seeking perfection but about tuning in to oneself as the first step to connecting with the rest of the world. Throughout life, challenges and deviations may lead us away from our inner being, but by recognizing our perfect nature and accepting circumstances with understanding, we can begin to transform our emotions and feelings.

By educating the mind, we can learn to direct our attention to the present, avoiding sadness over the past or anxiety about the future. Staying in the present allows us to connect with our internal source of energy and find peace in the present moment. Additionally, love plays a crucial role in life, as it can enhance quality of life by filling every part of the body with joy and tranquility, enabling us to face difficult moments with strength.

The activation of the pineal gland may involve a series of goals and potential benefits, although it is important to note that these may vary according to individual beliefs and practices. Some possible objectives of pineal gland activation could include:

1. **Emotional well-being**: Pineal gland activation could be associated with increased mental clarity, emotional balance, and a sense of inner calm.

2. **Sleep improvement**: It has been suggested that pineal gland activation and melatonin production may contribute to higher quality sleep and regulation of the circadian rhythm.

3. **Spiritual connection**: For some individuals, pineal gland activation is linked to greater spiritual perception, intuition, and awareness of dimensions beyond the physical.

4. **Expansion of consciousness**: Some practices related to pineal gland activation aim to expand individual consciousness and sensory perception.

5. **Health and vitality**: It has been suggested that the activation of the pineal gland may positively influence overall health and physical well-being, although this claim may vary and require further scientific research.

It is important to remember that pineal gland activation may be part of spiritual, philosophical, or alternative therapies, and that the results and benefits associated with it may vary depending on individual needs and experiences. If you are considering pineal gland activation, it is crucial to seek professional guidance and fully understand the potential benefits and risks involved.

The activation of the pineal gland involves exploring our emotions and recognizing the energy that surrounds us, including connection with nature, the sun, and the stars. It is a journey that deserves to be undertaken with professional guidance and expertise.

When the pineal gland is activated, a person may experience a variety of physical and mental effects, including:

Physical:

* Increased mental clarity and concentration

* Improved memory and cognition

* Greater energy and vitality

* Enhanced sleep regulation

* Reduction of stress and anxiety

* Heightened intuition and spiritual connection

* Decreased pain and inflammation

Mental:

* Altered states of consciousness

* Increased creativity and inspiration

* Deep sense of peace and serenity

* Connection with the higher self

* Visionary or mystical experiences

* Enhanced extrasensory perception

* Sense of purpose and direction

It is important to note that these effects can vary greatly from person to person and may not occur in all cases. Pineal gland activation is a gradual process that may take time and effort.

Personally, I underwent pineal gland activation with Cristian Vidal, who has over 23 years of experience in this and other types of therapies. This experience has been fundamental in my life, as I previously found it difficult to understand certain connections I felt with the sun, the moon, trees, water, etc. Also, when experiencing sadness, it used to linger for a long time, and learning to recognize that this emotion arises from the loss of something valuable, and that it has a very low vibration, has allowed me to address it more consciously. On the other hand, I have learned that anger is a normal and healthy emotion, as it is a natural response to perceived threats, but it is important to have control over it instead of being carried away, and that it only lasts for 3 minutes, the rest is just a show. These are just some of the learnings I have acquired with this professional, who is a wonderful human being full of wisdom and love.

85

Chapter 8

What is Intravenous Therapy?

"Always seek balance,

knowing your body

and nourishing your mind"

Intravenous therapy, also known as IV therapy, is a treatment that involves the intravenous administration of customized solutions designed to meet the specific needs of each individual in order to improve their well-being, health, and physical appearance. This therapeutic approach not only enhances the body's defense mechanisms but also promotes detoxification, regeneration, and repair.

By providing the body with a variety of nutrients, vitamins, and minerals directly and rapidly, intravenous therapy helps optimize bodily functions. It is important to note that this therapy can be beneficial regardless of the stage of the disease, and it can even be used in advanced cases such as cancer.

The human body tends to encounter various toxins, such as viruses, parasites, toxic metals, environmental pollutants, pesticides, medications, and even negative emotions and past traumas. Intravenous therapy offers the possibility of detoxifying the body, which is essential for aging with quality of life and well-being. Thanks to current scientific advances, achieving a pain-free life enriched by quality is feasible.

Intravenous therapy offers the application of personalized detoxifying solutions, following an evaluation of the body's toxicity level and considering the patient's medical history. This approach not only maintains but also restores and transports the necessary nutrients for the body.

Bioregulation, an active biological process induced by therapeutic intervention, has the ability to optimize and restore the body's self-regulation mechanisms. In addition, intravenous administration of solutions aims to normalize the physiological characteristics of the internal environment, especially the extracellular fluid surrounding multicellular cells.

The goal of intravenous therapy is to reduce the need for oral medication administration and polypharmacy. It also aims to maintain and restore plasma or circulatory volume, and serves as a route for the administration of substances such as medications, nutrients, and diagnostic elements.

Methylene blue has been studied for its potential effects on the brain when administered through intravenous therapy.

Its ability to act as a potential neuroprotective agent has been investigated, as well as its possible role in improving cognitive function and regulating various biochemical processes in the brain. However, it is important to note that the use of methylene blue for therapeutic purposes in the brain should be supervised and administered by qualified healthcare professionals, as its application and dosage must be carefully controlled to avoid adverse effects.

Methylene blue has also been researched for its potential to improve mitochondrial function, reduce free radical toxicity, and participate in the regulation of the immune system. Additionally, its potential for the treatment of mood disorders and depression has been studied.

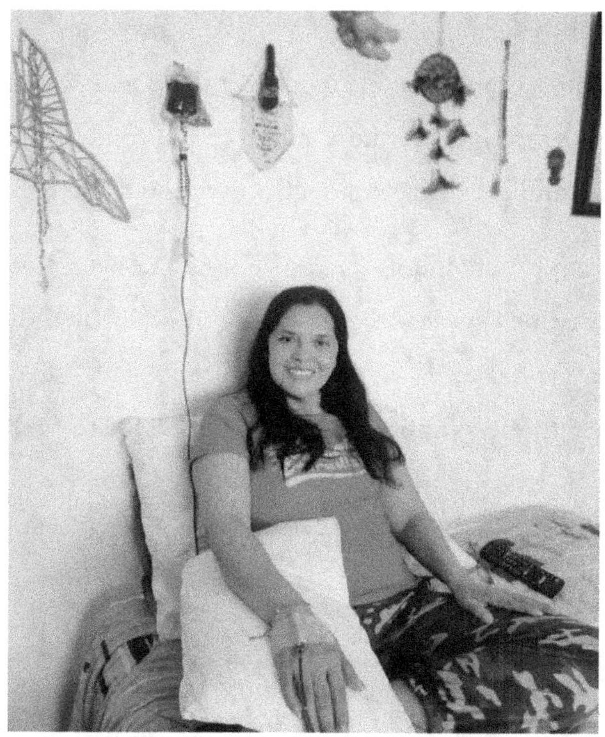

Calm and relaxed while receiving Methylene Blue intravenous therapy.

Non-invasive Intravenous Therapy (Micronebulization)

Another non-invasive form of intravenous therapy is Micronebulization, which provides a more inclusive approach; seeking a less complex, more comfortable route for both the individual and therapist, rapid, effective, and more natural.

Nebulizer solutions are devices that convert liquids into aerosol or fine droplets so that they can be inhaled through a mask or a nozzle. This allows medications to be delivered directly to the respiratory tract and lungs, which is particularly useful for treating respiratory conditions such as asthma, chronic bronchitis, COPD, and other lung diseases.

Nebulization is beneficial for several reasons:

1. By nebulizing a medication, it reaches the respiratory tract directly, which may result in a quicker action of the drug compared to oral or parenteral forms that require absorption and systemic distribution.

2. High Local Concentrations: Inhaled medications can reach higher concentrations at the desired site of action (the lungs), with less likelihood of causing systemic side effects.

3. Faster Onset of Action: Absorption of medications through the lungs is rapid, allowing for a quicker onset of

action, an important consideration in emergency situations such as acute asthma attacks.

4. Fewer Side Effects: Since the dose of the medication may be lower than the oral or parenteral form to achieve the desired therapeutic effect, there are potentially fewer side effects.

As for trace elements, they are of great importance in medicine and nutrition. Although they are needed in smaller amounts compared to other nutrients like macronutrients (proteins, carbohydrates, and fats), trace elements fulfill essential functions such as:

- Enzymatic cofactors: Many trace elements are components or cofactors of enzymes essential for biochemical processes.

- Maintenance of protein and cell membrane structure: Some are necessary to maintain the structural integrity of proteins and cell membranes.

- Regulation of gene expression: They have a role in regulating the expression of certain genes.

- Bone health and connective tissue formation.

They are found in many foods and are typically consumed through the diet, but there are situations where deficiencies or increased needs may justify supplementation.

Nebulization of solutions containing trace elements may be a mode of administration in very specific contexts; generally under the guidance of a healthcare professional, to treat deficiencies or disorders where inhalation of these elements may be beneficial. However, it is important for such treatments to be supervised due to the precision required in trace element doses and the potential toxicity in case of overdose.

Nebulized solutions are effective because inhaled drugs are deposited directly in the respiratory tract, resulting in high concentrations, with a faster onset of action and fewer side effects than if the systemic route is employed.

Trace elements are chemical components, elements that form living matter, and also participate in organic processes. Their concentrations are minimal and are generally found in food. Such as:

Magnesium is an essential mineral that plays a crucial role in numerous bodily functions, including supporting the nervous system, muscle function, bone health, blood sugar regulation, and protein and energy production.

Zinc is necessary for the immune system, wound healing, DNA metabolism and cell division, reproductive health, and the sense of taste and smell.

Potassium is an important electrolyte for fluid balance, muscle, nerve and heart function, and blood pressure.

Cobalt is a component of vitamin B12, essential for red blood cell formation and nervous system function.

Manganese is necessary for connective tissue formation, thyroid function, and bone structure.

Calcium is critical for bone and dental health, muscle contraction, blood clotting, nerve transmission, and heart function.

Chromium plays a role in blood sugar regulation and the metabolism of carbohydrates, fats, and proteins.

Iodine is essential for thyroid function and brain development during pregnancy and infancy.

Lithium is a mineral often associated with mental health and is used in the treatment of certain mood disorders.

Molybdenum is necessary for the function of certain enzymes and proper nutrient metabolism.

Iron is essential for red blood cell formation and oxygen transport in the body.

Silver, although not an essential nutrient, has traditionally been used for its antimicrobial properties and for other medicinal purposes.

Selenium is a key antioxidant that also plays a role in thyroid function and the immune system.

Phosphorus is necessary for bone and teeth formation, energy storage, and DNA and RNA production.

Sulfur is a critical component of amino acids and plays a role in skin, hair, and nail health.

Nickel, boron, silicon, vanadium, and germanium, although found in small amounts in the body, may have specific roles in metabolism and cellular health, although their exact role is not fully understood.

Sodium and copper are important for fluid balance, nerve transmission, and various enzymatic functions.

Overall, each of these minerals and trace elements performs unique and fundamental functions in the human body, contributing to health and optimal functioning of different physiological systems and processes.

"This therapy has proven to be effective for the administration of vitamin C and other nutrients, offering wonderful results. Personally, it helped me relieve dryness in the nasal passages. It is important to note that I do not intend to formulate anything in this book. I simply wish to share that these therapies exist and, when used in conjunction with a professional, can provide relief or even cure various discomforts in the body and mind".

Not all laboratories have medications for this therapy.

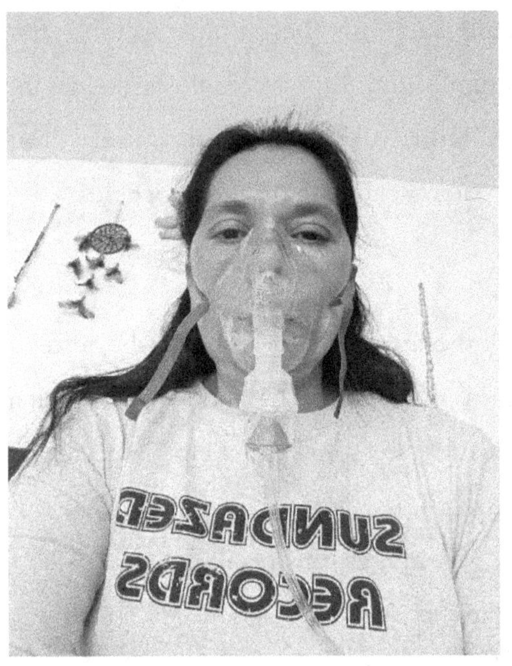

There are other complementary therapies not mentioned because there is not deep knowledge about them and I have not practiced them either.

Here are some of them:

1. Acupuncture: A traditional Chinese practice involving the insertion of thin needles into specific points on the body's skin to relieve pain and treat various health conditions.

2. Homeopathy: Based on the principle that "like cures like," homeopathy uses highly diluted substances with the aim of triggering the body's natural ability to heal itself.

3. Chiropractic: Focused on the diagnosis, treatment, and prevention of musculoskeletal disorders and their effect on overall health, often through spinal adjustments.

4. Aromatherapy: Use of essential oils extracted from plants to promote physical and psychological well-being, often through massage or air diffusion.

5. Therapeutic Massage: Manipulation of the body's soft tissues to reduce stress and pain, improve circulation, and promote relaxation.

6. Reflexology: Massage technique involving applying pressure to specific points, especially on the feet, believed to be related to other organs and systems of the body.

7. Reiki: Japanese-origin "energy healing" practice in which the therapist channels energy to the patient to stimulate the natural healing process.

It is important to mention that while some people find great benefit in these therapies, the scientific evidence of their effectiveness may be limited or vary widely depending on the specific therapy. It is always recommended to consult with a healthcare professional before starting any complementary therapy, especially if you have any pre-existing health conditions or are taking medication.

Chapter 9

What is Naturopathy?

"Always seek the path

towards natural healing,

and inner balance"

Naturopathy is a system of alternative medicine that focuses on the use of natural and holistic approaches to promote health and well-being. Practitioners of naturopathy, known as naturopaths, employ a variety of therapies and methods including herbal medicine, nutrition, homeopathy, acupuncture, massage, therapy with medicinal plants, and lifestyle counseling, among others.

The philosophy of naturopathy is based on the principle that the body has the innate ability to heal itself, and by providing a healing environment and supporting the body's natural processes, health can be restored and maintained optimally.

Naturopaths often work with their patients to identify and address the underlying causes of illnesses, rather than simply treating symptoms in isolation. Disease prevention, patient education, and promotion of a healthy lifestyle are also key elements of naturopathic practice, combining natural therapies such as nutrition, exercise, herbal therapy, and detoxification techniques with a belief in the healing ability of nature.

An expert in this field, such as a naturopathic doctor, may work with individuals suffering from a wide range of health issues, from acute conditions to chronic diseases. Some common approaches a naturopathic expert may use to support health and well-being include:

* Diet and nutrition counseling to address nutritional imbalances and promote gastrointestinal health.

* Use of medicinal herbs and natural supplements to support overall health and address specific issues.

* Detoxification therapies to help the body eliminate toxins and promote cellular health.

* Physical therapies such as acupuncture, massage therapy, and hydrotherapy to alleviate pain and promote relaxation.

* Self-care and stress management approaches, which may include breathing techniques, meditation, and therapeutic exercise.

Naturopaths may work with individuals suffering from a wide range of health conditions, including but not limited to:

* Digestive disorders, such as irritable bowel syndrome, indigestion, and diarrhea.

* Immune system issues, such as allergies and food sensitivities.

* Hormonal imbalances, such as premenstrual syndrome (PMS) or menopause.

* Stress, anxiety, and sleep disorders.

* Chronic pain, such as back pain or joint pain.

* Skin problems, such as acne, eczema, and psoriasis.

* Weight and nutrition-related issues.

* Chronic diseases, such as type 2 diabetes and high blood pressure.

It is important to remember that naturopathic therapy is not intended to replace conventional medical care; a naturopathic expert may work collaboratively with other healthcare professionals to provide a comprehensive and complementary approach to healthcare.

Naturopathy invites us to rediscover the ancient art of healing, in harmony with nature and in balance with our inner being, towards comprehensive and lasting health.

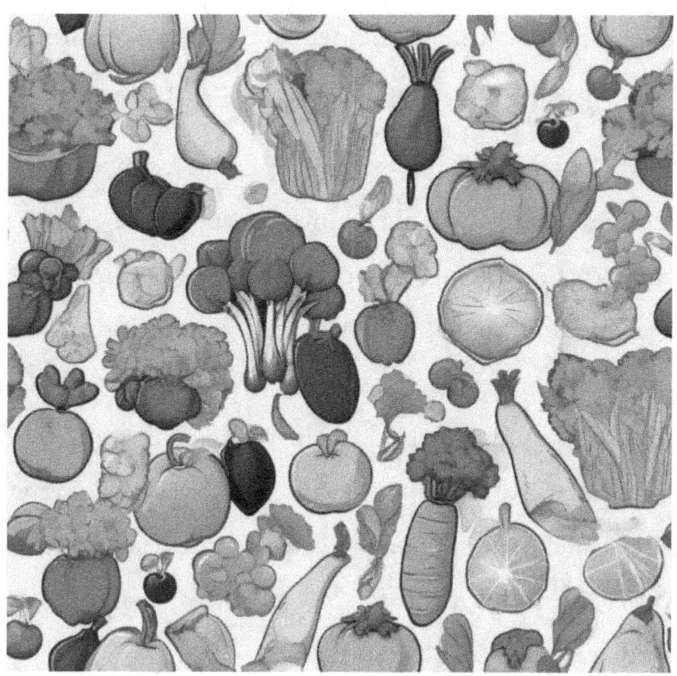

Chapter 10

Preparing the Subconscious Mind

> "The subconscious mind is like the hidden engine
> that drives our actions and thoughts without us being
> fully aware of it"

The subconscious mind is a part of the mind that is not currently in the focus of consciousness but still influences a person's behavior, actions, decisions, and feelings. It is considered to harbor memories, intuitions, automatic feelings, and thoughts that are not immediately accessible to consciousness but can spontaneously arise or be brought to consciousness through specific stimuli or introspection.

Although the subconscious operates below the level of conscious awareness, it plays an important role in our daily functioning. For example, it can influence our relationships, what we believe about ourselves, our motivations, and even our physical reactions. Psychology and other disciplines related to the study of the human mind explore methods to better understand and work with subconscious content to promote well-being and personal development; your subconscious mind is a source of ideas, aspirations, and altruistic needs for each person.

There are always two sides in life: subjective objective, visible and invisible thought and manifestation of it, the subconscious mind does not argue, it only acts according to what you write on it; we are always writing in the book of life because your thoughts become your own experiences.

The subconscious mind is considered powerful for various reasons, especially due to its influence on a person's behaviors, emotions, and decisions, often without the person being fully aware of that influence. Here are some of the "powers" or capabilities attributed to the subconscious:

1. Programming of behaviors and habits: Many of our daily habits and automatic reactions are managed by the subconscious. With repetition and practice, certain behaviors become automatic, freeing our conscious mind to focus on tasks that require more attention.

2. Storage of memories: The subconscious stores memories and past experiences. Although we may not always be able to consciously retrieve all this information, it can influence our present reactions and decisions.

3. Effortless information processing: Our subconscious processes information from the environment even when we are not actively paying attention. This can help us perceive

and react to situations without needing significant conscious effort.

4. Repair and healing during sleep: It is considered that, during sleep, especially in certain phases, the subconscious works on healing and emotional and physical readjustment, processing experiences and conflicts.

5. Intuition: Sometimes, the subconscious provides us with "hunches" or intuitions. These feelings may result from unconsciously processing information, leading us to conclusions that we could not have reasoned consciously.

6. Creative visualization and manifestation: Some theories and practices suggest that by positively and intentionally visualizing, we can program our subconscious to work toward those goals or desired states, thus affecting our motivation and conscious actions towards those ends.

7. Influence on bodily functioning: It is suggested that the subconscious can influence involuntary bodily functions and the healing process. Examples of this include the placebo effect or the manifestation of physical symptoms due to psychological causes.

However, although the subconscious has these capabilities, it is important to remember that its influence is intricately connected and cannot be completely separated from conscious awareness and other aspects of our psyche and brain functioning.

Moreover, the subconscious mind is always working day and night, whether you are walking or resting. It is important to keep the conscious mind busy with perspectives of the best, making sure your thoughts are based on love, truth, justice, and good deeds. Start taking care of your conscious mind because the subconscious mind is always reproducing and manifesting according to your frequent thoughts.

I want to share a story about how we can impress the idea of perfect health on our subconscious mind. This story was revealed to me by a priest in a clinic, while I was waiting for instructions for my next chemotherapy session. We were both there for similar reasons: me, preparing for my treatment, and him, with his test results in hand. In that moment of vulnerability, we shared unconventional healing methods, and he recounted his experience to me:

He strived to reach a state of deep relaxation, both physically and mentally, speaking to his body with soothing calmness. 'Everything in my body is relaxed: my feet, my knees, my heart, my liver, my lungs, my head, my whole being,' he would say to himself. After a few minutes of stillness, he would affirm with conviction: 'The image that God has of me is perfect; therefore, subconscious, reconfigure my body in accordance with that divine image.' The remarkable thing about his case is that, against all odds, the priest experienced a miraculous recovery.

This experience teaches us that our minds have immense power over our physical well-being, suggesting that by infusing concepts of health and perfection into our subconscious, we can influence our healing process.

I have talked to you in this chapter about the subconscious mind because if we put it into practice together with the therapies mentioned earlier, it is a wonderful duo, capable of restoring your health in body and mind in a more effective way.

The brain: It is a universe in constant expansion, where each thought is a new star that illuminates the infinite of our possibilities.

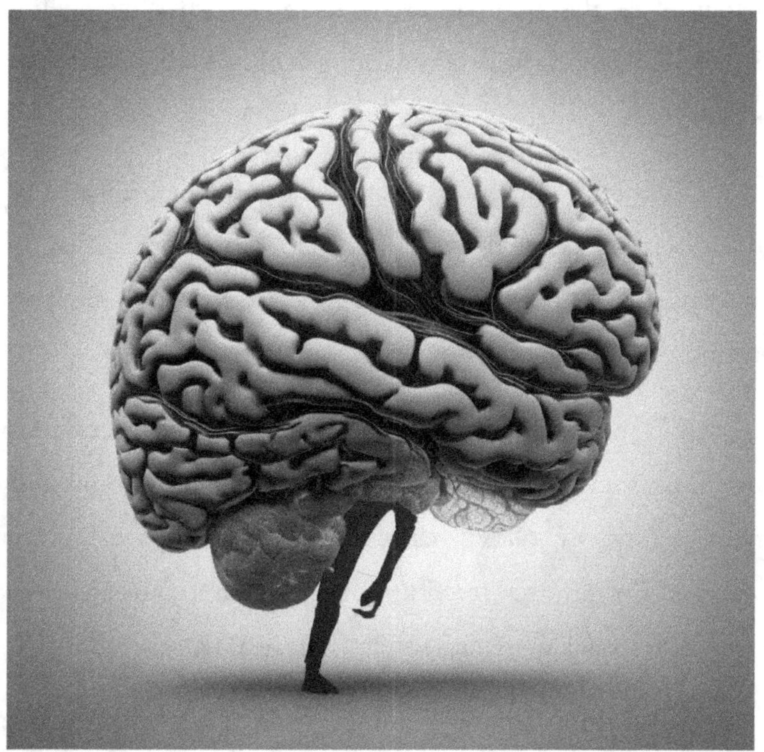

On the other hand, since we've talked about the subconscious mind, I also want to say something about the importance of not silencing our thoughts and letting them flow:

In the incessant journey of life, we often encounter thoughts and emotions that seem to overwhelm our mind and heart. In those moments of internal turmoil, it's easy to succumb to the temptation to suppress what we feel, to silence our deepest reflections out of fear of what they might reveal.

But aren't our thoughts and emotions the bridge to our true essence? Aren't the currents of our being the ones that guide us to a deeper understanding of ourselves and the world around us?

We should not fear our own thoughts, however dark or unsettling they may seem. On the contrary, we should allow them to flow, to follow their course like waters seeking their channel. For in the freedom of expressing our ideas and feelings lies the key to authenticity and healing.

So, do not fear your thoughts, do not silence them or relegate them to oblivion. Let them shine in your mind like stars in the night, illuminating your path and showing you the truth that resides deep within your being. Let your thoughts speak, let your emotions guide you, and you will discover the magic of being completely yourself in a world that sometimes urges us to be silent.

May the voice of your thoughts resonate in the vastness of your being, reminding you that in the freedom of expression and in the power of authenticity, you find the true essence of life. Let them pass, let them flow, and discover the beauty of being who you really are!

When the mind is filled with thoughts and you find yourself overwhelmed without knowing what to do, I recommend seeking refuge in nature and the company of animals. Take a moment to observe a majestic tree, an animal playing in the water, or simply the dance of dry leaves carried by the wind. You will realize that those thoughts that previously disturbed you have been left behind, allowing you to find tranquility in the present.

Conclusion

From the preceding discussion on complementary therapies, it can be said that we do not have eternal life; we can only live it. Therefore, we have an obligation to always seek for our body and mind to be in a state of stability in every sense, enabling us to walk the path that life presents to us with carefreeness and by getting closer to nature to heal ourselves.

Moreover, it doesn't matter the degree to which any illness is present; attempting to practice alternative medicine and all the therapies described here is always worthwhile. All of these have a common denominator, which is to heal body, mind, and spirit through all the nutrients existing within our bodies, which, for various reasons, cease to be produced naturally, such as imbalanced nutrition, toxic medications, environmental pollution, and lack of physical movement (exercising our bodies).

Recognizing who we are and where we want to go is essential to begin identifying the gaps, sufferings, and situations of the past that have been holding us back. Often, we carry superficial baggage that prevents us from moving forward, avoiding facing our weaknesses and fears. However, if we make the decision to confront these things with determination, we will realize that we were magnifying problems that were not really so serious. By giving them so much value, we were creating unnecessary resistance.

I am sure that every person is extraordinary inside; you should never stop being children and remember that there is nothing to fear or defend, only to walk the path; may it give us more enthusiasm, freedom, and moments of joy.

Everything natural will always be the best for restoring, nourishing, and accelerating our improvement in everything related to mental and physical health.

Identifying in time what causes certain behaviors in people makes it easier to work on them and thus solve said imbalance satisfactorily. Here is a unique opportunity to acquire valuable knowledge and strategies that can help minimize the suffering of various diseases. Seeking the cause is the most important thing.

On the other hand, from my perspective, the subconscious mind operates in a fascinating and complex way, influencing our lives in deep and unexpected ways. Through patterns, ingrained beliefs, and memories, the subconscious shapes our decisions and perceptions powerfully, often without us being aware of its influence. Recognizing and understanding this hidden part of our mind can be key to personal growth and transformation.

I have written this book with love, and I offer it to you, dear reader, with the hope that the suggestions offered here become a guide to seeking self-healing and your continued well-being, and to lead a full life, seeking the appropriate person to carry them out.

"Always seek positive answers to things that seem terrible"

In each book, I leave a writing for my son, who passed to another plane or whose energy changed.

"Death is simply the next great change in our existence, the step into the unknown that gives depth and meaning to our finite life in this world"

Ivan

Although you are no longer here by my side,

your love and courage have remained.

Your departure left a void in my being,

but it also gave me the strength to be reborn.

Every day I feel your spirit in my walk, guiding me with love, unceasingly.

Your absence is painful, it's true,

but your light accompanies me in the darkness.

You are the inspiration that fills my being,

a force that propels me to relive.

In every heartbeat, in every breath,

you remain present, infinitely.

I will honor your memory with love and passion,

living a life full of compassion.

Your departure taught me to be brave,

and with you, son of my heart, it will be forever.

"Contemplate with gratitude the mystery and beauty of nature, a gift that gives us life, sustenance, and refuge on our journey through this existence. In every tree, in every river, in every animal, resides the essence of creation, a reminder of our duty to love, respect, and protect our mother earth"

I invite you to immerse yourself in the wisdom of nature, to connect with its healing and transformative power. May every leaf, every breeze, every bird song inspire you to take care of our common home, to be guardians of the life that sustains and nourishes us. Let's live in harmony with nature, honoring its greatness and protecting its fragility!

SOCIAL MEDIA

117

https://www.youtube.com/@magalydiazb

https://www.facebook.com/magadiazbarrios/

https://www.instagram.com/magadiazbarrios/

www.ingramcontent.com/pod-product-compliance
Lightning Source LLC
Chambersburg PA
CBHW071040250726
48653CB00005B/1919